The Pocketbook of
Positivity and Reframing

The Pocketbook of Positivity and Reframing

Fifty reminders, including practical tips, on how to be positive and to reframe what might seem like negative situations into opportunities for growth

Pauline Ronan

www.stepforward-coaching.co.uk

This book is dedicated to my beautiful family, who have allowed me to dream, and to all my beautiful friends, who have indulged my endless discussions on being mindful, meditation, positivity and the power of reframing.

Contents

About the author 1

How to use this book 6

Introduction 8

1 Being a true friend to yourself 12

2 Loving the warts and all 14

3 Matching success patterns 16

4 Planning to sleep well 18

5 Pass on the good vibes 20

6 Self-love and kindness 22

7 Catching self-doubt 24

8 The power of sleep 26

9 Breathe in a new day 28

10 Awe and wonder 30

11 Working through strong emotions 32

12 What can you do for others today? 34

13 Be the observer and reduce the pain 36

14 Checking our reaction 38

15 You do not always have to know the answer . 40

16 Patience is a virtue 42

17 Mind your language 44

18 The happiness recipe 46

19 See the bus 48

20 Growing amidst the suffering 50

21 Engage the brain 52

22 Cultivating our garden 54

23 Addressing the feelings...........................56

24 Reframing the 'failures'..........................58

25 This is me!..60

26 Thank you for today 62

27 Mindfulness as medicine........................64

28 Trusting our inner teacher 66

29 What is your inner soundtrack?............68

30 Fighting the demons...............................70

31 My own best friend 72

32 Choosing our mindset for the day 74

33 Dissatisfied moments are good teachers 76

34 Milestones...78

35 Finding joy in the everyday mundane.............80

36 Finding peaceful moments 82

37 Celebrate the story in every scar...........84

38 The basic beauties are the best 86

39 Recognising the fleeting feeling 88

40 The choice is yours 90

41 Deal with the facts..................................92

42 Looking for the 'good seeds' 94

43 Being nurturing to yourself during change.....96

44 Inviting the creativity to flow...............98

45 The niggling voice................................100

46 Checking your thoughts 102

47 Choosing your reaction wisely............104

48 Are you listening to me? 106

49 What message am I giving to my brain? 108

50 My imagination 110

A final thought ~ The power of exercise 112

References 119

About the author

About six years ago, I was feeling lost, stuck and unsure of my direction. How could it be that I had a successful job, a great family, a lovely husband and son, but I was no longer sure who I was anymore?

I knew there was more to be had. I did not want to be on the side-lines anymore. I really wanted a change and an exciting new purpose, but I did not know what I was looking for. I wanted to grow into my own skin and feel connected and fully alive as my own best friend. I wanted to offer myself kindness and compassion. I wanted to feel good and look good from the inside out, but I had to find the tools to make these ambitions a reality.

As I mulled over these desires, I decided it was time to make a change. I began to explore yoga and meditation to see if they could help me find out who I was and what I was missing. I had to think hard about what I actually wanted out of life and what I needed to do to move forward.

My journey really began when I spent some time

having a deep personal reflection and started to self-nurture. I began to understand the connection between my thoughts, my body and the emotions I was experiencing. I found that I could take simple baby steps that would allow me to blossom into the woman I wanted to be.

I observed those around me who had positive attitudes, especially in difficult situations, and realised they got the best outcomes and often lived happier and healthier lives. I read constantly about how we can change our mindset for the better. I developed an understanding of who I was and why I was feeling less joyful. The more I learnt and understood, the more I felt empowered and uplifted and that anything was actually possible.

I was excited to learn that by reframing scenarios in a positive way I could feed my brain a positive message instead of having the negative soundtrack playing in my mind. An ingenious but very simple trick! The imagination is such a creative tool, but I realised that it can also enable you to waste time creating imaginary negative scenarios in your head that might never happen. I started to explore information about the brain and found out how the amygdala, our gatekeeper, will react to situations in a fight or flight mode. I soon discovered that by recognising that we are in the moment, we can slow these reactions down and change the outcome from a potential drama to a fleeting moment.

By putting all that I learnt into practice I became so much happier, more vibrant and, most importantly, I was becoming me again. My family and friends started to notice a positive change. I had found my voice once more. I had developed the confidence to make exciting changes without the fear of failing. Now I was ready to make a few more changes with the help of my internal introspection.

With my new lease of life, I made the decision to start running, which released the serotonin and endorphins in my brain and helped me feel good. I returned to that enthusiastic and curious person who wanted to experience more and enjoy life to the full. With my new running routine, I was delighted to find I was able to lose a stone in weight and I started to feel fantastic. Running also opened connections to my local community and allowed me to meet so many lovely new friends. In 2018, I ran my first marathon which felt like a pivotal moment in this truly incredible journey.

I started to think about how I could use my new-found knowledge and enlightenment to help others. I realised just how many people, particularly women, felt like I had—lost and unsure. I realised that sharing positivity and using reframing could help people to move forward quite quickly, instead of lingering in the same repetitive and negative story over and over.

I am now very happy to say that I am a qualified life coach and well on my way to being a Human Givens Psychotherapist. I also have my own coaching business called 'Step Forward Coaching'. My work allows me to encourage people to move forward with a big emphasis on exercise, meditation and visualisation. I love what I do and feel delighted that I can help an individual to transform and blossom by enabling them to access their own inner toolbox.

If you are feeling any of the same emotions that I did, I really hope that this book will inspire you to change the angle on your view. This book will help you to realise that there are exciting opportunities out there for you to grab with both hands, and that there is nothing to be afraid of.

Let the next chapter commence in your life!

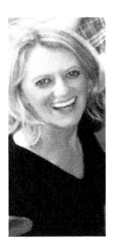

Pauline is Irish born and lives in Crosby, Liverpool with her husband, son and dog. Pauline returns to Ireland every six weeks to see her parents and five sisters.

How to use this book

If I was buying this book for my friend, I would encourage them to have it close by them every day, in their handbag, in their briefcase or on their desk. It might be the first thing that they read when they wake up or the last thing that they read at night. They might choose to keep it in the glove compartment in their car and have a quick peek at it before or after a meeting.

Each time you read one of the teachings it is a fresh reminder to be mindful and to see each day as an opportunity. It might not be a perfect day, in fact it might feel like a disaster, but by reframing situations you can flip it around and see the benefits.

If it is a major life event, it might not feel good at that time and it may take a few hours, days or weeks to calm down, but when you look at the event through a positive set of eyes, it can be such a good learning tool. Also, the way that we react is pivotal to our positivity, and practising non-reactive behaviour has benefits in abundance not just for your relationships, but also for your health.

With each daily teaching you have an opportunity to highlight parts of the text that you connect with on that day. You might like to date it, and when you come back to it at a later stage, you might realise how quickly thoughts come and go and can change.

I hope that you enjoy this book, that you buy one for your friends and that using it becomes a good habit.

£1 from your purchase will go to Papyrus, a small UK charity who campaign for suicide prevention. They remind us that there is always something to live for, even if it is not always clear in that moment.

Introduction

The really good thing about life is that you can always change your way of thinking. Every day that you wake up you have a choice. Dr Carol Dweck (2012) writes extensively on the benefits of a 'growth mindset', but you do not have to be born that way, it is a habit that you can form. Aristotle (350 BCE) talks comprehensively about virtue ethics.

A virtue is a characteristic that someone has, like honesty and integrity, but likewise the virtue of positivity. These virtues can be cultivated and developed. Aristotle teaches us that in order for a character to be developed it must be practised, so just like builders build to become better builders, guitar players play often to become a better guitar player, likewise optimists practice optimism and positivity to be optimistic.

Optimists are the best people to be around. They are unfazed by challenges and, in fact, relish them. Optimists are constantly looking for opportunities to grow and develop, even if it is tough. Optimists enjoy a challenge and have a deep belief in their ability to master a situation. An optimist will always see the half glass full and will be determined to try again.

This does not mean that it is easy to be an optimist, it takes lots of hard work, passion and a strong mind, but it is within us all. Optimists are more resilient. They make better entrepreneurs, experience better health outcomes, live longer and are more satisfied with their relationships (Medina, 2017). Optimism enables people to continue to strive in the face of difficulty, while pessimism leaves them depressed and resigned to failure—even expecting it.

I have been truly fortunate to have read many beautiful books and listened to many podcasts, particularly over the course of the last few years. One poignant book I read was *The Choice* by Dr Edith Eger (2017). Part of the book discusses the harrowing account of what she believes were her final moments in Gunskirchen Lager, the subcamp of Mauthausen, Austria. Her reflections have stayed with me since, as the positivity, although it would seem incredibly hard to find, is there in the most unlikely of places. It is particularly striking, as Edith and her sister Magda lay in the forest surrounding the death camp waiting to be extinguished, the whole place was rigged with dynamite, ready to be destroyed by the Gestapo.

As Edith lies there, surrounded by numerous bodies, death and decay, thoughts run through her head, some lucidly, others not so much, but she still has hope. She still manages to have hope when the liberators arrive at the camp, on that particular day. She dreams of being seen, even though she cannot talk anymore, but her fight has not left her. The American liberators shout 'raise your hand if you are alive', Edith tries to move her fingers, to signal she is alive but to no avail, she is not seen and the liberators are leaving presuming that nobody is alive.

Then a patch of light explodes on the ground. At first Edith thinks it is the fire that she has been anticipating from the exploding dynamite. The soldiers turn, the gleam of light is not fire at all, it is the sun colliding with Magda's sardine can, that she has been holding since it was donated by the Red Cross but with no way of opening it.

The soldiers are returning, this is now one more chance of freedom. Edith thinks, if I can dance in my mind, I can make my body move and be spotted. By some bizarre stroke of luck, the soldier touches her hand and realises she is alive. She is saved.

This account reminds us that even in the darkest of moments in our lives, there is still hope, something to be salvaged, something to be learnt and something to live for. We are not going to get over huge life events quickly, in fact we may never get over them at all, but we can learn to live with them, finding moments of understanding and of gratitude for the smallest of things.

Today, make a choice. Am I going to practice optimism in whatever form I can manage? It will benefit you, the individual; it will benefit your relationships; it will draw more optimism your way and ultimately it will make you happier, as you will be choosing to live as the best version of you. ▢

1

Being a true friend to yourself

Hopefully, everyone has a good friend that they can think of. They might be fully present in your life now or may have been a large part of it in the past. That good friend is the one who makes you feel great about yourself, is a tonic to be around and lifts your thinking.

Today, when harsh self-criticism comes into your mind, which is inevitable for us all, think of that good friend. That voice should be a soothing, compassionate voice in your head, showing you love and kindness.

Tap into this voice regularly and tell the harsh critic to be quiet. This selective self-talk can turn your thinking and your day around.

Notes

www.stepforward-coaching.co.uk

2

Loving the warts and all

It can be exhausting striving to be the best version of ourselves in our relationships, our work, our goals, our family or wherever else you make this effort.

True, self-improvement is crucial to our development, but some days it is important to 'just be' here in the moment, warts and all.

Today, visualise self-acceptance and remember that you are enough, just the way you are.

Notes

_____

_____

_____

_____

_____

_____

_____

_____

_____

_____

_____

_____

_____

_____

_____

_____

_____

www.stepforward-coaching.co.uk

_____

3

Matching success patterns

When we start something new like a job, a relationship, a new chapter of some sort, it can be incredibly daunting. We often experience self-doubt and frustration with ourselves, thinking why cannot these new skills come naturally or happen faster?

The easiest way to deal with this is to return in your mind to a previous success. What did you do previously? How did you get there? How did it feel when it was achieved?

Success is transferable, and the principles that you applied then can be applied repeatedly

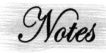

www.stepforward-coaching.co.uk

4

Planning to sleep well

If you are waking up in the middle of the night with things on your mind, have a notepad at the side of your bed to jot down the thing that might be bothering you.

Do not take time to analyse it or ruminate about it, just purely observe its appearance in your mind.

When you lie back down to sleep, begin to do a body scan, observing the parts of the body from the head through to the toes, using the breath as an anchor, count to 7 as you breathe in and 11 as you breathe out (Griffiths and Tyrell, 2013).

All the things in the notepad can be dealt with or thought about the next day.

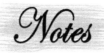

5

Pass on the good vibes

Remembering our intention today is to self-nurture and restore. When we are kind to ourselves through our thoughts and actions, we become so much kinder to those around us. We are less irritable, more accepting of others and their habits.

We also become very clear on how we want to be treated and give off a vibe that we matter and are important, not in an arrogant way, but in a gentle and loving way.

Today, use that loving kindness that you are extending to yourself and pass it on to others. You might pay for someone's coffee, send flowers to a friend who needs cheering up or write a letter to a loved one.

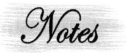

www.stepforward-coaching.co.uk

6

Self-love and kindness

Today should be a day of gentleness and kindness to yourself.

Delicately allow yourself lots of tenderness, not taking on harsh thoughts or judgements, moving slowly and with lots of self-love and nurturing, whilst sending good thoughts to others.

Notes

_____

_____

_____

_____

_____

_____

_____

_____

_____

_____

_____

_____

_____

_____

_____

_____

_____

_____

_____

www.stepforward-coaching.co.uk

_____

7

Catching self-doubt

When we start our day, our body naturally starts to worry about the tasks ahead and what is in the news. Our usual self-doubts can start playing their soundtrack in your head—but catch yourself in this ruminating moment.

Look at this day as an opportunity. Reframe what seem to be negatives as possibilities. Approach the day with acceptance and calm and get ready to have a day filled with gratitude, maybe even a smile.

Every day is a chance to learn and be fully awake, even if what lies ahead is tough.

Notes

8

The power of sleep

Sleep is not a luxury; it is a necessity. When we sleep it is divided into two parts: one is called slow-wave sleep and the other is called dream-sleep (Griffiths and Tyrell, 2013). Both parts are as necessary as the other, and when we do not sleep properly then sleep cannot function the way that it is intended to.

When you go to bed tonight, turn off all electronics a few hours in advance. Avoid any deep or angry conversations prior to sleep. Eat three hours in advance and maybe read a good book to help you to drift off.

When you wake, remind yourself that your actions during the day are just as important as the preparation before bedtime.

Notes

9

Breathe in a new day

Today, when you inhale, breathe in confidence, self-belief and positivity. See the good in situations, new choices and new freedoms.

When you exhale, let go of all those tensions that do not serve you well—doubt, lack of self-belief, negative self-talk and worrying about what others think of you.

Breathe in with possibilities and breathe out the negatives. This short exercise can change the way you approach your day.

Notes

10

Awe and wonder

Today, we think about our environment. As we work through the kindness we show to ourselves and others, we become aware of the beauty around us.

Maybe today you can feel the grass or sand beneath your feet, look up at the sky, maybe appreciate a sunset whilst remembering that you are part of this universe, with all its beauty and complexities.

Notes

11

Working through strong emotions

When we experience strong emotions such as anger, loss, fear and doubt, it is really easy to get swept away and caught up in the story. However, the more we are aware of our emotions and reactions, the more we can control them and control how they physically affect us.

When emotion arises, using the acronym RAIN is really beneficial (O'Morain, 2019). This means **recognising** the emotion that is there. **Acknowledging** the emotion, for example 'fear is here', not running away from it. **Investigating** what you can do to solve it, then **nurturing** and wrapping yourself in gentle compassion.

Be your own best friend and, of course, breathe.

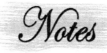

_____

_____

_____

_____

_____

_____

_____

_____

_____

_____

_____

_____

_____

_____

_____

_____

www.stepforward-coaching.co.uk

_____

12

What can you do for others today?

Today, try and remember that humans are inherently good. One way to be really fulfilled, as a human, is to be kind to ourselves and contribute to the community around us. You might be doing that already in your job or in your own home.

Why not write a letter today to someone who needs it, pick up the phone to someone, leave something for your neighbour or donate to a charity?

Helping other people makes us feel better and takes us out of our own mind, remembering we are better as a community (Aristotle, 350 BCE). Plus, the small, inexpensive acts are normally the most powerful of all.

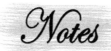

www.stepforward-coaching.co.uk

13

Be the observer and reduce the pain

When we recall an embarrassing or painful memory, as you think about it, it is normally so painful because you are seeing it through your own eyes. The intensity is greater because the experience is being relived through your own eyes repeatedly.

Now try and see the same situation as an observer. See yourself standing there experiencing the moment. Turn the lights down on the image in your mind and make the image smaller. Do it again. Make the image smaller again.

Keep on repeating this process and each time you return to the memory, it will appear smaller and smaller and eventually less significant and less painful (Bandler, website).

Notes

14

Checking our reaction

Accepting events as they are helps us to slow down reactions and prevents catastrophising. Life won't always go as planned, but we can say to ourselves when something unplanned or sad comes our way, 'this is where I am at right now'.

By using this phrase, we allow ourselves to sit with the problem, not reacting to it, just recognising it is there. Straight away this gives us back control.

As we are not fighting the feeling, we are giving ourselves this peaceful time for answers to come, and with them, solutions.

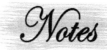

www.stepforward-coaching.co.uk

15

You do not always have to know the answer

Today, remember that it is okay to not know what will happen next. It is okay to not have all the answers or know everything.

For a few minutes today, just sit with the moment, without having to problem solve. Just be. Count to 7 as you breathe in and to 11 as you let go (Griffiths and Tyrell, 2013).

The longer exhalations relax the parasympathetic nervous system, helping you to enjoy the moment.

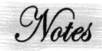

_____

_____

_____

_____

_____

_____

_____

_____

_____

_____

_____

_____

_____

_____

_____

_____

_____

_____

www.stepforward-coaching.co.uk

_____

16

Patience is a virtue

Today, try and practice patience. Patience with ourselves, patience with others, like our loved ones or friends, and most importantly, patience with situations.

Bringing patience to our daily mindfulness practice translates to the other parts of our lives. For example, when we want something done faster, want a queue to move quicker, or feel frustration with ourselves for not being able to achieve a goal more immediately.

Patience can teach us wisdom. Take the time to sit back and observe instead of going straight in and getting annoyed, letting things unfold in their own time. Then ask, 'what can we learn whilst we wait?'

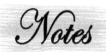

17

Mind your language

Today, take time to think about the language you are using. Are you presenting something in a really negative way? For example, 'I can't move jobs, as I can't do anything else.'

If you change it to 'I am really excited and looking forward to having a new challenge', it puts such a different spin on exactly the same message. You are telling your brain that this is possible, rather than presenting a barrier or an excuse that may stop you from being truly happy.

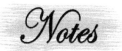

18

The happiness recipe

Happiness does not happen by chance, it normally takes hard work, determination, continual goal setting and bundles of positivity and hope.

What could you do differently today or how could you approach a problem in a new way to achieve happiness for yourself?

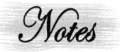

19

See the bus

Today, if feelings such as anger, frustration or sadness arise, simply observe them. Do not react to them, just notice that they are there. If we react to them, it can cause a spiral of events, maybe saying things in the heat of the moment and regretting it later.

So today, imagine thoughts are like buses. They frequently pass you by, just like thoughts. You do not have to get on every bus you see. Similarly, you do not have to attach yourself to every thought you have. Recognise them. Acknowledge them. Remember that is all they are, thoughts. As quickly as the bus comes, it is gone, just like our fleeting thoughts (Headspace app).

Always remember the anchor point for your breath, maybe it is feeling the breath in your nostrils, chest or tummy. Think of the word 'returning'. This practice ultimately slows down our emotional brain, the amygdala, and enables us to manage our feelings and reactions much better.

Notes

20

Growing amidst the suffering

In life, whether we like it or not, there is suffering, such as bereavements, divorce and illness, and there are setbacks scuppering all the original plans we had in mind.

You might think, 'Why is this happening to me?' You might think, 'That's not how it was meant to be.' Those thoughts are natural and human.

However, suffering and setbacks help us to grow and transform. Instead of pulling the duvet over your head and hoping that these pains go away, face your hardships with courage and gentleness, remembering that this time of pain will pass.

If we allow ourselves the space to grow, knowing that hope will get us through, everything will be okay and we might be a bit wiser at the end of it, even if it looks different to what we had originally hoped for.

Notes

21

Engage the brain

Sometimes the idea of gratitude and kindness is a hard one, especially when tough times and challenges are coming at us thick and fast.

Being grateful and kind is actually good for us and can often bring us to a better and happier place. In fact, some emotions engage the left side of our brain, so neurologically they have benefits, as they lift our mood.

Maybe today spread some kindness to a loved one, someone you have not spoken to in a while or even extend that olive branch to someone who has wronged you, being grateful for the simple things that we do have.

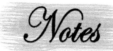

22

Cultivating our garden

Daily mindfulness is the idea of being in the moment, not ruminating in the past or being fretful about the future. Putting one foot in front of the other and appreciating this moment, right now.

Mindfulness is a great habit to cultivate and, just like tending to a garden, we must look after it fully in order for it to grow and develop. A tree does not just appear. The soil needs to be prepared and enriched.

Just like patience and acceptance does not just appear in us, we must practice good habits daily, in a disciplined way, for these traits to form and stay with us, and then we will prosper fully.

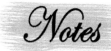

23

Addressing the feelings

When we have feelings that we are not happy with, we think they are going to last forever, but usually a few hours or days later the feeling moves on.

Remember to observe the feeling, knowing that it will pass. Some problems might have to be solved and addressed when the time is right, which is part of life.

The observation of the feeling without reacting is the most crucial part of mindfulness. It might even be useful to write it down.

Notes

24

Reframing the 'failures'

It is so tempting, when we have spare time, to start ruminating about what is not right in our lives and past 'failures', but when those memories arise, plant your feet firmly on the ground, count to 7 as you breathe in and 11 as you breathe out (Griffiths and Tyrell, 2013), reminding yourself 'this is where I am at right now'.

Maybe when the time is right, return to the memory and reframe what seems like a failure. What has that experience taught you, what are the positives of what seem like a mistake? You never know, that situation or scenario may have taught you invaluable skills or developed resources you did not think you had.

Notes

_____

_____

_____

_____

_____

_____

_____

_____

_____

_____

_____

_____

_____

_____

_____

_____

www.stepforward-coaching.co.uk

25

This is me!

Perfection is accepting ourselves, flaws and all, which creates the fabric of you!

Remember that comparison is the thief of joy.

Notes

26

Thank you for today

One of the best ways to get happiness to come your way is to have gratitude.

At the beginning of each day or each evening, set five minutes aside and go through up to ten things that you are grateful for. For example, you woke up this morning, you can read this message, you have a bed to sleep in and hopefully you can feel love and are loved.

The list can be seemingly endless, but during this time of appreciation, if we allow joy to enter our hearts, it puts a smile on our face and reminds us that when things seem bleak there are so many things to be grateful for.

Notes

27

Mindfulness as medicine

Some cynics think that mindfulness is a wishy-washy concept and are wary of it. Mindfulness is the idea of being in the moment, not ruminating in the past or being fretful about the future.

When we are mindful, the left part of our brain engages the amygdala, our emotional brain, which calms us down and makes us less reactive. The NHS recommends mindfulness to reduce feelings of anxiety and feeling depressed; plus, it helps us to really relish the good parts of life. So today, allocate some time to be mindful, maybe when you are cooking, eating, brushing your teeth or walking.

Feel the ground beneath you and focus on your breath using the 7–11 technique (Griffiths and Tyrell, 2013), count to 7 as you breathe in and 11 as you breathe out. You are engaging the parasympathetic nervous system by breathing out longer, which may be in turn makes you more patient and less irritable around those you love.

Notes

28

Trusting our inner teacher

'Everything that came before had to happen to us to be the person we are now. The greatest moments of clarity come when we look back and we realise it was all necessary' (Hawker, 2015).

What can we learn from personal circumstances? What situations have actually enabled us to grow as people as a result of that testing time? Recognise that situations, both good and bad, are always there, ready to teach us about our own inner resources, some of which we did not even realise we had.

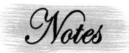

29

What is your inner soundtrack?

Some people listen to the same story in their own head for years about past hurts, injustices and regrets. Are these unresolved issues actually serving you?

This morning when you wake up, remind yourself that 'this is where I am at right now'. Become aware of your breath. Maybe notice it mostly in your nostrils, your chest or your tummy. Place both feet flat on the floor and think of one thing you are grateful for.

Welcome to now, not yesterday or tomorrow, just this moment, right now, accepting the good and the more challenging parts.

Notes

30

Fighting the demons

Our worries are all linked to the emotional brain called the amygdala. It derives from prehistoric man who believed that when we are in fight or flight mode, ultimately our body prepares for survival (Griffiths and Tyrell, 2013).

It is unlikely we will be chased by a tiger today, but we might need to handle our own demons, those little voices in our head that cause us anxiety. Our emotional brain reacts when we recall a painful memory or when we are afraid of a future scenario.

Our imagination runs wild and that is when we get those anxious feelings in our stomach, throat and chest as we rehearse worst case scenarios in our head.

Maybe today, if you find yourself in that moment, just breathe. Keep your feet flat on the ground. Be aware of any sensations in the body. Mindfulness can help reduce worry.

Notes

31

My own best friend

The person who needs to be your best friend is you. We need to treat ourselves with compassion and love, like we do our partner, children and friends. Sometimes this involves lots of self-acceptance and at times, humour.

So, the next time you have negative, berating self-talk in your mind, think, 'Is this what I would tell my child, partner or best friend?' Self-love is not selfish, it is crucial.

Notes

32

Choosing our mindset for the day

When we wake up in the morning, we might think about all the things that are good or about all the things that are bad. Sometimes it is much easier to think of the bad and draw people into our negativity, which usually becomes unproductive.

This morning, focus on what is good. Tell other people about it. Share the positivity around and you will get it back in abundance. There are good and bad things in life, that is a fact, but how we react to them is always a choice.

Now tap into a little inner smile and let's face the day well.

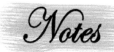

33

Dissatisfied moments are good teachers

Often, we are so intent on pursuing the end goal, for example, a new career, a 10k run or moving house, that when something gets in our way, it just becomes annoying.

That thing getting in the way could be here to teach us something vital about what really matters, about what we are like as individuals. It might be here to help us recognise that there will be times of dissatisfaction, but that is okay.

Consider the next dissatisfied moment which comes your way. What can you learn from it? Can you accept it? Is it not just part of your fabric, your story? It is not just the end goal that is important, it is the journey to get there.

Notes

_____

_____

_____

_____

_____

_____

_____

_____

_____

_____

_____

_____

_____

_____

_____

_____

www.stepforward-coaching.co.uk

34

Milestones

As we reach the end of the day, week or month, take a moment to reflect on what you have achieved so far. Maybe by yourself or with friends and family.

If you have been worrying, catch yourself doing it and consider, 'Could it be reframed in a different way or could I act to change it?'

As Mark Twain said, 'I've had some terrible experiences in my life and some have actually happened.' Much of our fear is in our own mind (Twain, Good reads website).

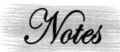

_____

_____

_____

_____

_____

_____

_____

_____

_____

_____

_____

_____

_____

_____

_____

www.stepforward-coaching.co.uk
_____

35

Finding joy in the everyday mundane

Things that might seem boring or mundane do not have to be negative. Having positive thoughts whilst doing everyday jobs, like washing the dishes, keeps us optimistic.

During these moments we can notice the sky outside our kitchen window or glance at a photograph of loved ones or our favourite places. Reframe what might seem like 'hassle' as opportunities to be still and to savour the here and now.

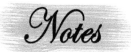

_____

_____

_____

_____

_____

_____

_____

_____

_____

_____

_____

_____

_____

_____

_____

_____

www.stepforward-coaching.co.uk

36

Finding peaceful moments

Sometimes when we do nothing we feel guilty that we are not running around keeping busy with our daily routines. Difficult as this may seem, we should give ourselves a day that is just neutral. Not filled with moments of sadness or joy, just ordinary.

Sometimes 'ordinary' is just ideal. Peaceful, still and drama-free.

Notes

37

Celebrate the story in every scar

This is our really big challenge, to grow into our own skin, warts and all. Accepting that each scar and line tells a story, accepting all the aspects with compassion and honesty.

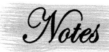

38

The basic beauties are the best

We spend so long as humans chasing 'stuff'—the nicest holidays, the cars, the clothes—but actually when it boils down to it, the best things in life are free, like hugs, chats, laughs together with family and friends, or a Sunday roast dinner around the table.

So maybe today catch yourself appreciating some of those basic beauties and treasure them.

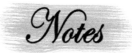

39

Recognising the fleeting feeling

Recognising how we feel right now is powerful, but not reacting to the feeling is even more powerful.

Thoughts are like buses, we can observe them driving around in our mind, but we do not have to get on them and take a seat. Just recognise that they are there and then in a flash, they are gone.

We are not ignoring them, just not reacting to them in that moment. We come back to them when the time is right, when we have the energy and wisdom to deal with them.

Notes

40

The choice is yours

In life, although it does not always feel that way, we have a choice. A choice to be happy, a choice to have a positive mindset, a choice to say yes or no.

Your first duty of care is to yourself. Make your wellbeing a priority, always remembering to put your own oxygen mask on first.

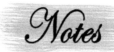

www.stepforward-coaching.co.uk

41

Deal with the facts

What might start off as a small resentment or niggle can grow into something huge and consuming if you allow it. A comment or an action can be interpreted and over-exaggerated, and if you give it enough airtime, it can become your soundtrack, the thing you listen to, day in and day out.

Our brain interprets situations, and that is natural, but remember to 'deal with the facts' first before jumping to conclusions or negative speculations, which can increase anxiety and concern.

Today, if your mind wonders about a resentment or niggle, come back to being in the moment. Deep breaths in and long breaths out, feet flat on the floor, and when you are ready, ask yourself, 'What are the facts?'

Notes

42

Looking for the 'good seeds'

During tough days we still need to look for the 'good seeds', taking time to appreciate the good things in our situation, today and in our life. Watering the 'bad seeds' is ruminating on what is wrong in our life, our faults and failings.

Finding the 'good seeds' is not always easy but it leads to a much better balance and a happier individual, helping you to step out of the gloom.

Notes

43

Being nurturing to yourself during change

When we have to adapt to a big change in our lives, if it is not what we are used to or is not particularly easy, we must always show ourselves self-compassion. Once we do this, it extends to everyone else around us, allowing more harmony to exist.

Gradually over time and with patience, the new becomes the norm. Learn to do this through meditation and being mindful throughout the day.

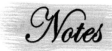

www.stepforward-coaching.co.uk

44

Inviting the creativity to flow

Today, we focus on being creative and expressive. Today might be your day to start writing down how you are feeling, fears, uncertainties, delights and things to look forward to.

You do not need any fancy language, just a way for you to offload. You might do this through a letter, a poem, a piece of artwork, or starting to dance or sing.

When we meditate or are mindful, we allow for space and with space comes creativity.

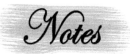

_____

_____

_____

_____

_____

_____

_____

_____

_____

_____

_____

_____

_____

_____

_____

www.stepforward-coaching.co.uk

45

The niggling voice

Everyone has an inner dialogue, that is natural, but the voice we use in our head can build us up or knock us down.

Try self-compassion today, being kind to yourself even if vital changes have to be made. Ask yourself, 'Is the voice mine or somebody else's?' Try changing the voice to a comical one, with a different accent and the impact of the comments is not as damaging (Bandler, website).

Notes

46

Checking your thoughts

Today, when you are doing everyday things such as brushing your teeth, sitting in a work meeting, doing housework or exercising, think to yourself, 'Are my thoughts healthy and productive?'

Start to become aware of your thinking patterns. Are you worrying about future events, letting your imagination run away with you or imagining worst case scenarios that might never actually happen?

Check in with your thoughts regularly, come back to the breath, the constant anchor, with your feet flat on the floor, count to 7 as you breathe in and 11 as you breathe out. The only moment you have for certain is now (Griffiths and Tyrell, 2013).

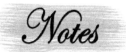

www.stepforward-coaching.co.uk

47

Choosing your reaction wisely

During incredibly challenging times, our reactions become everything.

Remind yourself that feeling peaceful is a much nicer feeling than feeling angry.

Use the mantra 'this is where I am at right now' to bring a level of acceptance.

Notes

48

Are you listening to me?

Today, try to actively listen. When our families and friends or work colleagues talk to us about something, look at them in the face, ensure that your phone is out of sight and really listen.

Try not to think about what you are going to say next, or interrupt them, or try and fix their problem with a solution, just listen. When they are finished, pause. This pause tells them that you are listening and might give them the space to say more.

Repeat some of the things they have said, reiterating that you are listening whilst building rapport. The more we actively listen, the better listeners we become.

Notes

49

What message am I giving to my brain?

Remember, what you focus on, you get. The brain is a pattern-matching organ and whatever pattern you focus on, the brain does its best to match it.

So, if you are constantly calling positivity to you through your thoughts and actions and having gratitude for your life, that is what you will get.

Likewise, if you are calling negativity to you and sending out negativity and being mean to yourself and others, do not be surprised if you have a negative day or a long-term negative experience.

Remember, you can choose the messages that you send to your brain by the thoughts you have. Thoughts become things.

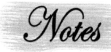

50

My imagination

Our imagination is our worst and best tool. At its worst, it can spin a simple situation and develop it into a massive fear, for example, if someone makes a comment, we could spend hours mulling over it, making judgements and twisting a simple phrase into a catastrophic interpretation.

In the same vein, our imagination is where dreams start. Every invention, book, song, poem, career change and new life stage started as a dream, and for the courageous became a delight. We have the choice every day.

Notes

A final thought
The power of exercise

Exercise is medicine.

Two hours of aerobic exercise a week is the equivalent to using antidepressants. Exercise increases blood flow to the brain and raises the levels of brain chemicals such as serotonin and dopamine. Higher serotonin levels make us feel good. Dopamine helps create a sense of motivation, which makes us feel good, too. (Griffiths and Tyrell, 2004). You can get this through running, walking, cycling, dancing, tennis or whatever you want as long as you are moving; plus, exercising in natural light, also releases serotonin.

My 'go to' exercise is running. My sister introduced me to running. When I first started, I would run a little bit and then walk, feeling out of breath. I would get shin splints and found it really tough. Despite this, I kept on going. Why? Because when I got home, I felt great. I felt energised. I would feel achy but happy. Things that had bothered me before I left the house seemed lighter somehow. I had a new lease of life and a natural high.

I am fortunate to live by the beach; it is stunningly beautiful. Every day is different. Some days are light and breezy whilst others are wintery, with crashing waves. This image is probably a good analogy of life as some days are lovely, while others are tough. You just have to keep going, though, in the knowledge that after the tough part, there is often sunshine, yet you cannot have the sunshine without the hard work and grit beforehand.

Three years into my running I got a running partner, our dog Goldie. She is a mix of Labrador, Golden Retriever and Collie. This triple combination makes her loyal, friendly and an avid runner, so my perfect companion. She does not make any demands of me, except that I rub her belly and give her hugs, which I can deal with.

Running has also opened up a social life like never before. I have met some of the most fantastic people through my local running clubs, especially my weekly parkrun, an ingenious idea devised by Paul Sinton-Hewitt.

My local parkrun in Crosby was initiated by the

wonderful Jan Mullin, an incredibly caring person who wanted to give others an outlet to exercise whilst connecting with people and building up self-esteem. The parkrun itself is a challenging run with three types of terrain: sand, tarmac and grass.

I had been running many 10k's and half marathons and my sister encouraged me to try a marathon. I wanted to see if I could, so I did. It was an incredible experience which I could tick off my bucket list, but it also taught me that I am a really happy 5k girl!

The best thing about the parkrun, though, is the volunteering opportunity. Having started to volunteer over the last few years, I enjoy nothing better than clapping people on with Goldie at my side. I always stand in the same spot. I repeatedly have a gulp in my throat every time someone shouts, 'Thanks, marshal'; these are people who might be regular runners, they might be fast or slow. They might be novices, trying to lose weight, wanting to look after their minds, or people who just need a bit of privacy to zone out for an hour of their day, and they are thanking me for turning up. It is an absolute privilege.

Afterwards, when we have collected all the

equipment and made sure all the runners are back safely, then we start with the tea and cake. The volunteers make cake to have afterwards and I have the fondest memories of chatting to people from all different backgrounds about a variety of topics. The joy of parkrun and volunteering! A genius plan, set up by Paul Sinton-Hewitt.

If exercise is not part of your routine, this might be the right time to make that change. You do not have to be fast or an Olympian, but you must have a desire to look after yourself. To keep your body strong so that you feel good about you. It is incredible how you can problem solve or tap into creativity through a short blast of exercise, and how life may look very different afterwards, particularly if you can fit better into your clothes!

Notes

_____

_____

_____

_____

_____

_____

_____

_____

_____

_____

_____

_____

_____

_____

_____

_____

_____

www.stepforward-coaching.co.uk

Notes

References

Aristotle. *Nicomachean Ethics.* Written 350 BCE.
Translated by W. D. Ross.

Bandler, Richard. Neuro Linguistic Program Training.
www.richardbandler.com

Dweck, Dr Carol. *Mindset: Changing the way you think to fulfil your potential.* Random House, 2012.

Eger, Dr Edith. *The Choice.* Penguin Books, 2017.

Griffiths, J. and Tyrell, I. *How to Lift Depression Fast.* Human Givens Publishing, 2004.

Griffiths, J. and Tyrell, I. *Human Givens: The New Approach to Emotional Health and Clear Thinking.* Human Givens Publishing, 2013.

Hawker, Lizzie. *Runner.* Aurum, 2015.

Headspace App

Medina, John. *Brain Rules for Aging Well.* Pear Press, 2017.

O'Morain, Padraig. *Daily Calm.* Yellow Kite, 2019.

Twain, Mark. Good Reads Website, www.goodreads.com, 2020.

Printed in Great Britain
by Amazon

35722026R00078